Livingood Health Habits

The Essential Guide to Everyday Well-being

David C. Radley

Copyright © 2024 by David C. Radley

This book is a work of nonfiction. Names, characters, businesses, places, events, locales, and incidents are either the products of the author's experience or used in a factual manner. Any resemblance to actual persons, living or dead, or actual events is purely coincidental.

While the author and publisher have made every effort to ensure the accuracy and completeness of the information conveyed in this book, they assume no responsibility for errors, inaccuracies, omissions, or any inconsistency herein. Any slights of people, places, or organizations are unintentional.

ACKNOWLEDGEMENT

As I think on the journey that led to the publication of "Livingood Health Habits: The Essential Guide to Everyday Well-Being," my heart is filled with gratitude for the many people who have illuminated the path along the way. This book is not just the result of my personal experiences and ideas, but also a tapestry weaved from the wisdom and assistance of others.

First and foremost, I want to honor the pioneering authors whose writings have served as beacons of knowledge and inspiration. To Michael Pollan, whose research into food and culture has transformed our understanding of nutrition; Deepak Chopra, whose integration of mind, body, and spirit has opened up new avenues for wellness; and Brene Brown, whose work on vulnerability and strength has taught us the value of emotional well-being. Their groundbreaking efforts have not only improved my life, but also sparked the idea for this book.

I'm also extremely grateful to my family, whose continuous support has been my rock. To my husband, whose patience and encouragement have been as steady as the northern star; to my children, whose zeal for life reminds me every day of the benefits of health; and to my parents, whose love and guidance have shaped the person I am today. You are my foundation, my biggest supporters, and my greatest blessing.

Thank you to my mentors and colleagues for challenging me, engaging in many discussions, and constantly pushing me to aim higher and dig deeper. Your intellectual generosity and collaborative spirit have proven beneficial.

I'd like to express my gratitude to the health and wellness community, including practitioners, researchers, and activists, for their relentless efforts to expand our understanding of health. Your commitment to the well-being of others is an ongoing source of motivation.

My readers, this book is for you. This guide exists because of your commitment to improving your health and the faith you have placed in these pages. May it be a useful tool on your road to everyday well-being.

Finally, to the unsung heroes—farmers, instructors, caregivers, and all those who nourish life in its varied forms—your contributions constitute the foundation of our civilization. You remind us that health is not a solo pursuit, but rather a collaborative symphony.

"Livingood Health Habits" exemplifies the common wisdom and shared human experience that unites us all. I acknowledge each of you with profound respect and gratitude.

CONTENTS

INTRODUCTION

Welcome to a Healthier You

Welcome to a Healthier You, the core of "Livingood Health Habits: The Essential Guide to Everyday Well-Being." This book is more than a collection of pages; it's a trip, a discourse, and a promise of change. It's where your journey to health and happiness begins.

Imagine waking up every day feeling revitalized, with vitality that lasts from the moment you open your eyes until you lie down to sleep. Consider a life in which well-being is not merely a goal, but integrated into the fabric of your daily existence. This is the life that "Livingood Health Habits" offers you to embrace—a life in which every day is an opportunity to nourish your body, mind, and soul.

As you go on this journey, you'll realize that health is more than just the absence of illness; it's a condition of total harmony between the body, mind, and spirit. It's about making decisions that promote your well-being and reflect your innermost values. Everything begins with the habits you establish on a daily basis.

This book will help you build those behaviors. It's a road map to a healthy you, complete with actionable guidance, evidence-based solutions, and compassionate encouragement. Every facet of health is studied, understood, and embraced, from the food you eat to the way you walk, from the quality of your sleep to the peace of mind you have.

You'll discover that nutrition is the foundation of health, supplying the fuel for all body functions. However, it is more than just eating less or more; it is also important to eat well. You'll learn about the concepts of a balanced diet, the value of whole foods, and how to navigate today's nutritional landscape.

Physical activity is also an important component of overall health. It strengthens the heart, improves mental health, and enhances life expectancy. Whether you're a seasoned athlete or just getting started, you'll discover strategies to incorporate various forms of exercise into your daily routine, regardless of your fitness level.

Restorative sleep is essential for wellness. It's time for the body to restore itself. You'll learn the significance of sleep quality, the stages of sleep, and practical ways for improving your sleep habits.

But health is more than just physical. Mental health is as vital. You'll look at stress management techniques, the power of positive thinking, and ways to build resilience and coping abilities.

Let us not forget the power of relationships. Humans are social beings, and our interactions with others have a profound impact on our overall health. This book emphasizes the importance of good relationships and community involvement.

Your environment has a wide range of effects on your health. You'll learn about environmental elements that influence well-being, such as air quality and noise levels, as well as how to build a healthy environment.

"Livingood Health Habits" also delves into integrative and alternative medicine, covering topics such as acupuncture, massage, and herbal therapies, as well as their possible benefits and drawbacks.

Self-care is the practice of actively protecting one's own health and pleasure. You'll learn how to create a self-care practice that is good for your body and mind.

As you flip each page, you'll find inspiring stories, informative information, and engaging activities. You will be challenged to think differently, take risks, and accept change. You will be encouraged at every stage, cheered on in every success, and guided through every failure.

This book is a celebration of health, a monument to the human spirit, and a light of hope for those seeking a more active life. It serves as a reminder that health is a journey, not a destination, and that each step forward leads to a better version of yourself.

So, take a deep breath and walk forth with confidence. Your journey to a better you awaits, and "Livingood Health Habits: The Essential Guide to Everyday Well-Being" is here to help. Welcome to your trip. Welcome to a healthier and happier self.

The Philosophy of Everyday Well-being

In the early morning, when the world is silent and the day is full of possibilities, you stand by the window, coffee in hand, pondering the voyage ahead. This is an excellent time to consider the philosophy of everyday well-being—a concept that is both ancient and urgently current, and one that "Livingood Health Habits: The Essential Guide to Everyday Well-being" throws into clear, actionable relief.

Imagine a life in which well-being is as natural as breathing, where health is not pursued via frenzied spurts of exercise or fad diets, but rather enjoyed moment by moment with joy and ease. This is the center of our philosophy, the spirit of this book, and the essence of the adventure you are about to take.

Everyday well-being is not a faraway summit to be conquered, but a route to be taken with purpose. It is found in the simple decisions you make every day—the food you consume, the air you breathe, the activities you love, and the relationships you value. It is woven into the fabric of your everyday life, not as a set of activities, but as a tapestry of habits that help and maintain you.

"Livingood Health Habits" will guide you down this path. It is a book based on the notion that well-being is multifaceted, embracing physical, emotional, mental, and spiritual components of existence. It acknowledges that health is deeply personal yet universally desired—a thread that binds us all together.

As you turn the pages, you'll discover inspiring stories, effective strategies, and timeless knowledge. You will learn how to nourish your body with energizing and delicious foods, how to move your body with strengthening and soothing activities, and how to rest your body with restorative and rejuvenating sleep.

However, this book is about more than the body. It's all about the mind—the thoughts that shape your world, the mindfulness that offers tranquility, and the learning that promotes growth. It is all about the heart—the love that connects you to others, the compassion that heals, and the thankfulness that uplifts.

And it is all about the spirit—the sense of purpose that propels you, the connection to something higher that gives life meaning, and the joy that comes from living in harmony with your authentic self.

This is the concept of everyday well-being: a life lived with purpose, a body cared for with knowledge, a mind enlightened with wisdom, a heart opened with love, and a spirit lifted with joy.

So take a deep breath. Move forth with boldness and curiosity. The journey to a healthy you begins right now, and "Livingood Health Habits: The Essential Guide to Everyday Well-Being" is here to help. Welcome to your fresh beginnings.

How to Use This Book

Imagine standing at the shore of a tranquil lake, a lovely breeze whispering through the trees and the water's surface reflecting the sky above. This is your time forrdt thought, to consider the path that lies ahead. "Livingood Health Habits: The Essential Guide to Everyday Well-Being" is your compass, guide, and constant companion on your path to a healthier, more vibrant you.

This book is more than simply a passive read; it's an engaging experience in which you engage with your deepest wishes for well-being. It's a guide who communicates directly to you in a language that's both straightforward and easy, but profound and transformative. It's a wealth of information, stories, and actionable activities that will guide, motivate, and inspire you to adopt the concept of everyday well-being.

The chapter "How to Use This Book" establishes the foundation for your change. It's where you'll learn to navigate the pages that come after, not just with your eyes, but with your heart and soul. This book is designed to be your personal wellness coach, providing ideas and exercises that are as entertaining as they are informative.

You'll begin by establishing your intentions, identifying what health means to you, and visualizing the life you want to live. Each chapter will build on the previous one, resulting in a complete approach to health that addresses your physical, mental, emotional, and spiritual well-being.

As you progress through the chapters, you will see that each one serves as a stepping stone to the next, with each notion adding depth and richness to your understanding of health. You'll learn about the four pillars of good health, the value of nutrition, the joy of activity, the rejuvenating power of sleep, and the deep impact of mindfulness and relationships on your well-being.

This book, however, is about transformation rather than simply providing information. It's about taking what you've learned and applying it to your life in useful, meaningful ways. It's about making modest improvements that produce large outcomes. It's all about finding balance, harmony, and joy in the everyday.

Each part is interactive, with contemplation prompts, practice tasks, and opportunities to document your thoughts and progress. You are encouraged to interact with the content, to question, reflect, and personalize the discoveries.

The tone of the book is encouraging and motivating. It's like having a supporting friend by your side who encourages you, believes in you, and reminds you of your strength and potential. It's a voice that says, "You can do this," even when the going gets rough.

And when you get to the end of the book, you'll discover that it's not the end at all. It marks the beginning of a new way of living and being. It's the beginning of a journey that will linger long after the final page is turned, one that you are now completely prepared to embark on with confidence and excitement.

So take a deep breath. Open your heart and mind. And let's start this trip together. Hello and welcome to "Livingood Health Habits: The Essential Guide to

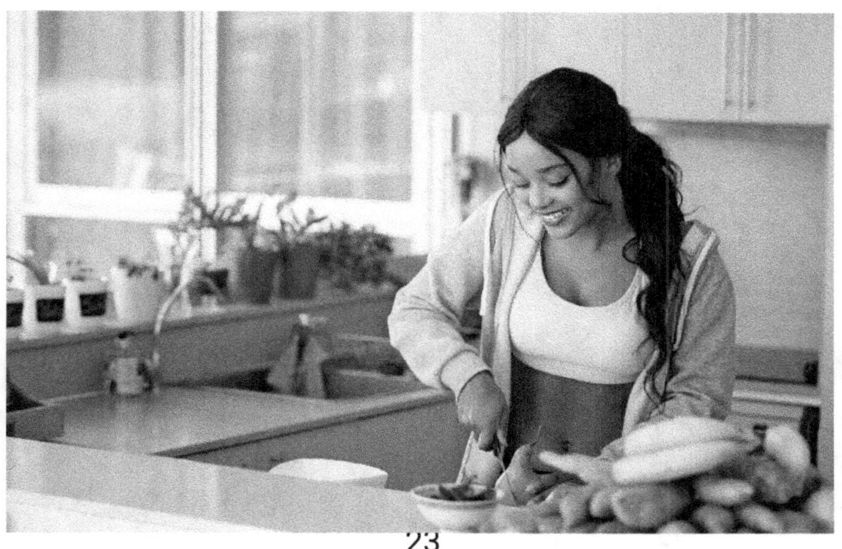

Everyday Well-being." Welcome to a healthier and happier self.

Part I: Foundations of Health

Understanding Health Beyond Medicine

Health is frequently defined as the absence of disease or weakness, but it includes much more. This chapter goes into the holistic approach to health, which includes the entire individual and how they interact with their surroundings.

The Bio-Psychosocial Model

We present the biopsychosocial model, which views health as a dynamic interplay of biological elements, psychological circumstances, and social pressures. This concept proposes that treating symptoms with medication is only one element of healing.

Nutrition: The Foundation of Physical Health

Investigate how a balanced diet delivers the nutrients required for the body to function properly. We'll talk about the roles of macronutrients and micronutrients, the significance of gut health, and how to make informed dietary decisions.

Exercise: Beyond Burning Calories

Physical activity is essential for preserving muscle strength, cardiovascular health, and mental well-being. Learn about the various types of exercise and how consistent movement can help prevent chronic diseases.

Sleep: The Unknown Hero of Health

Sleep is essential for recuperation, cognitive functioning, and emotional stability. This section discusses sleep hygiene techniques and common sleep disorders, emphasizing the need of good sleep.

Mental Health: Emotional Aspect

Mental health is equally vital as physical health. We'll look at stress management techniques, the benefits of positive thinking, and ways for building resilience and coping abilities.

Social Connections: The Fabric of Our Wellbeing

Humans are social beings, and our interactions with others have a profound impact on our overall health. This section discusses the advantages of good relationships and community involvement.

Environmental influences

Our environment affect our health in a variety of ways. We'll look at environmental elements that affect our well-being, such as air quality and noise levels, and how to build a healthy environment.

Integrative and complementary medicine

Discover alternative therapies to supplement established medicine. We'll talk about acupuncture, massage, and herbal therapies, as well as the potential benefits and drawbacks.

Self-Care: Your Personal Health Responsibility

Self-care is the practice of actively protecting one's own health and pleasure. We'll share advice on how to create a self-care practice that benefits both the body and the mind.

The Pillars of Livingood Health

Several pillars serve as the foundation for the route to good health. These pillars represent the most important characteristics of a healthy living. In this chapter, we will look at each pillar in depth, examining their roles and how they work together to create a healthy and vibrant life.

Pillar 1: Nutrition

Nutrition is the fuel that drives all of our body functions. It's not simply about eating less or more; it's about eating well. This section discusses the concepts of a balanced diet, the value of whole foods, and how to navigate the modern nutritional environment.

Pillar 2: Physical Activity

Regular physical activity is an essential component of healthy health. It strengthens the heart, improves mental health, and enhances life expectancy. We'll discuss how to incorporate several types of exercise into your everyday routine, regardless of your fitness level.

Pillar 3: Sleep and Rest

Restorative sleep is essential for wellness. It's time for the body to restore itself. This pillar stresses the importance of sleep quality, sleep stages, and practical ways to enhance your sleep patterns.

Pillar 4: Stress Management

Chronic stress can cause havoc in the body. This section offers stress-management tools and practices, such as mindfulness, breathing exercises, and time management measures.

Pillar 5: Hydration

Water is life. Proper hydration is essential for all cells in the body. We'll look at the science of hydration, how much water you need, and the role of electrolytes in maintaining fluid equilibrium.

Pillar 6: Social Connections

Humans are social organisms by nature, and our connections have a tremendous impact on our health. This pillar investigates the impact of social ties on health and offers suggestions for developing meaningful interactions.

Pillar 7: Mental Well-being

Mental health is equally vital as physical health. This section highlights the significance of mental resilience, emotional intelligence, and techniques to promote mental health through hobbies, therapy, and self-reflection.

Pillar 8: Environmental Health

Our environment has a huge impact on our health. We'll talk about how to build a healthy living environment, the value of interacting with nature, and how to reduce contaminants.

Pillar 9: Purpose and Passion

Living a life that is consistent with your values and passions is critical for your well-being. This pillar urges readers to discover their purpose and follow it with zeal, as alignment is a significant driver of health.

Nutrition: Fueling Your Well-being

Nutrition is the foundation of health. It provides our bodies with energy, serves as the foundation for our cells, and provides fuel for our well-being. This chapter delves into the enormous impact nutrition has on our lives and offers practical tips for sustaining your body and mind.

The Science of Nutrition

We begin with a review of nutrition science, discussing how the body processes various nutrients and their roles in health maintenance. We will cover:

- **Macronutrients:** Carbohydrates, proteins, and lipids, and their proportions in a healthy diet.
- Micronutrients are vitamins and minerals that play vital roles in biological processes.

- Phytonutrients are plant-based chemicals that offer considerable health advantages.

Eating for energy

Learn how to eat to maintain energy throughout the day. This section provides advice for balancing blood sugar levels with the proper foods.

- Understanding the Glycemic Index and its significance.
- Timing meals and snacks to improve metabolic health.

Gut Health: The Center of Your Universe

The stomach is often referred to as the second brain because of its impact on general health. Topics include the microbiome and its impact on digestion, immunity, and mood.

- What are probiotics and prebiotics, and how may they be included in your diet?
- The relationship between intestinal health and chronic disease.

Food as medicine

Discover how eating can help prevent and treat sickness. We'll talk about anti-inflammatory foods and their benefits.

- The link between diet and illnesses such as diabetes, heart disease, and cancer.
- Strategies for incorporating a healing diet.

The Art of Mindful Eating

Mindful eating entails being present with your food. This section addresses mindful eating techniques and their advantages.

- How to respond to your body's hunger and fullness cues.
- The psychological dimensions of eating and food selection.

Making Dietary Choices

With so many diet options available, it can be difficult to make the proper one. We'll investigate:

- Pros and disadvantages of popular diets like keto, vegan, paleo, and Mediterranean.
- How to customize your diet to meet your specific needs and goals.
- The importance of dietary variety and moderation.

Practical Nutrition

This section offers practical suggestions for incorporating healthy eating into your daily life, including meal planning and preparation tips.

- Healthy substitutions for everyday items.
- Tips for eating healthy on a budget.

Movement: The Joy of Being Active

Movement is a celebration of life. It expresses our vitality and demonstrates our ability to interact with the world. This chapter delves into the numerous ways in which being active benefits our health, happiness, and overall quality of life.

The biology of movement

We begin by discussing the basic basis of movement and how it affects the body. Topics include:

- The Musculoskeletal System describes how muscles, bones, and joints interact during physical action.
- **Cardiovascular Benefits:** Regular physical activity provides heart-healthy benefits.
- **Endocrine Response:** The role of hormones such as endorphins, which are produced during exercise and contribute to the 'runner's high.

Types of Physical Activities

Everyone can engage in some type of physical activity. We will cover:

- Aerobic exercises, such as walking, jogging, and swimming, help to enhance endurance.
- Strength training involves using resistance workouts to increase muscle and bone density.
- **Flexibility and Balance:** Exercises such as yoga and tai chi can improve joint health and avoid falls.

Exercise and Mental Health.

Physical activity is an effective strategy for mental health. This section discusses how exercise can relieve anxiety and depression.

- How activity might boost cognitive function and memory.
- The social benefits of group exercise and sports.

Finding Your Movement

Finding an activity that you enjoy is essential for incorporating movement into your daily routine. We'll talk about how to experiment with different types of exercise and determine what works best for you.

- The value of diversity in keeping your routine interesting and difficult.
- Strategies for incorporating activity into your regular routine despite a hectic schedule.

Overcoming Barriers to Exercise

We explore common barriers to regular physical activity, including time limits and strategies for managing them.

- Physical constraints and how to deal with them.
- How to overcome a lack of motivation and discover inspiration.

Setting Goals and Tracking Progress

Setting goals might help you stay motivated and live an active lifestyle. This component contains:

- How to set SMART (Specific, Measurable, Achievable, Relevant, and Time-bound) fitness objectives.
- The advantages of tracking progress and rewarding achievements.
- Utilizing technology, such as fitness trackers and apps, to aid in your path

Sleep: Restoring Body and Mind

Sleep is not a passive condition, but rather a dynamic process that is necessary for our physical and mental recovery. This chapter explores the transforming impact of sleep and offers ways for maximizing its restorative benefits.

The Science Of Sleep

Understanding sleep starts with the science behind it. We'll investigate:

- **Sleep Cycles:** The various stages of sleep, including REM and non-REM, and their importance.
- **Circadian Rhythms:** How our internal clock regulates sleep patterns, and the consequences of disturbing them.
- **Sleep Hormones:** How melatonin and other hormones regulate sleep.

Benefits of Quality Sleep

Quality sleep is a key component of wellness. This section emphasizes the multiple benefits:

- **Physical Health:** How sleep promotes healing, growth, and illness prevention.

- **Mental Clarity:** How sleep affects cognitive activities such as memory, learning, and decision making.
- **Emotional Regulation:** The relationship between sleep and emotion, particularly how it helps to manage stress and anxiety.

Common Sleep Challenges

Many people battle with sleep disorders. We'll discuss common issues like:

- Understanding insomnia's causes and discovering viable therapies.
- **Sleep Apnea:** The health concerns connected with the illness and potential treatment options.
- **Restless Leg Syndrome:** What it is and how to get relief.

Creating A Sleep-Conducive Environment

The environment greatly influences sleep quality. Tips for creating a sleep-friendly environment include:

- **Lighting:** The necessity of darkness and how to control light exposure.
- **Noise:** How to reduce noise pollution and use soundscapes to relax.
- **Temperature:** determining the best temperature for sleep and the advantages of a cool sleeping environment.

Sleep hygiene practices

A good night's sleep is dependent on proper sleep hygiene. This portion provides practical advice:

Routine: Creating a consistent sleep pattern to help your circadian rhythm.

- **Diet and exercise:** How your eating habits and level of physical activity effect your sleep.
- **Relaxation techniques:** Meditation, deep breathing, and progressive muscular relaxation can all help you get ready for sleep.

Technology & Sleep

In the modern world, electronics can disrupt sleep. We will discuss:

- **Screen Time:** Blue Light's Effects on Sleep and Electronic Use Guidelines.
- **Sleep Trackers:** How to utilize technology to track and improve your sleeping habits.

Special Considerations

Sleep requirements differ during the lifespan and between individuals. We'll discuss how children and teenagers have different sleep needs.

- **Shift Work:** Coping strategies for folks who work non-traditional hours.
- **Aging:** Understanding how our sleep habits vary with age and how to adjust.

Part II: Building Your Livingood Habits

Hydration: The Essence of Vitality

The cornerstone of every temple of health is hydration. Water is needed for proper operation of every cell, tissue, and organ in our body. The main focus of this chapter is on how to successfully include drinking enough of water into our everyday routines and how important it is to preserving energy.

The Part Water Plays in the Body

Every living process takes place through water. Participating in it are:

- **Transportation:** Getting oxygen and nutrients to cells.
- **Control:** Sustaining other homeostatic processes and the body temperature.
- **Lubrication:** Smooth joint movement and tissue protection.

Understanding Dehydration

You become dehydrated when you use up or lose more fluid than you intake. We'll look at:

- Symptoms and Indications Knowing the early indicators of dehydration, include thirst, dark urine, and exhaustion.
- The health effects of persistent dehydration, both short- and long-term.
- Populations in Peril Finding those at greater danger, such as athletes, the elderly, and youngsters.

Just How Much Water Do We Actually Need?

Though the "8x8" rule—eight 8-ounce glasses of water a day—is well-known, everyone's needs are different. Within this section are covered:

- **Factors Influencing Hydration Needs:** Diet, environment, health issues, and degree of exercise.
- **Hydration Indicators:** Acquiring the ability to read your body's cues and interpreting urine color.

Water Goodness

Every water is not made equally. Discussed will be:

- Sources of Water Distilled, mineral, spring, filtered, and tap water.
- Potential contaminants and ways to make sure your water is safe to drink.
- **Improving Hydration:** Electrolyte function and natural replenishment methods.

Eating to Hydrate

Drinking water alone does not make one hydrated. We consume fluids in many foods. Ideas covered include:

- **Foods High in Water:** Watermelons, oranges, and cucumbers.
- Adding salads, smoothies, and soups to your diet will help you stay hydrate.
- Juggling Consumption of Food and Fluids: Recognizing the ways in which various foods can impact hydration states.

Sports Hydration

The hydration requirements of athletes are special. This section offers information about: Pre-Exercise Hydration: Getting your body ready for the demands of exercise.

- **Hydration While Working Out:** Understanding the Warning Signs and How to Remain Hydrated.
- **Post-Exercise Rehydration:** Effective strategies for replenishing fluids and electrolytes.

Water and Control of Weight

A healthy weight can be maintained in part by drinking enough water. Checked out will be:

- **Appetite and Fullness:** How the consumption of water can modify sensations of hunger and fullness.
- **Metabolic Rate and Energy Expense:** The Effect of Hydration.
- Debunking myths and laying out the facts about water intake and fat loss.

Everyday Hydration

Building hydration habits is vital for prolonged well-being. This section offers:

- **Daily Hydration Tips:** Practical techniques to boost your water intake throughout the day.
- **Hydration Tracking:** Tools and approaches for tracking your fluid consumption.
- **Overcoming Barriers:** Addressing frequent problems to staying hydrated, such as forgetfulness and aversion of plain water.

Special Considerations

We handle specific conditions that necessitate attention to hydration, such as:

- **Illness and Recovery:** The increased requirement for fluids during sickness.
- **Travel:** Staying hydrated on long journeys and in varied climes.
- **Aging:** Adjusting hydration tactics as we grow older.

Mindfulness: The Art of Presence

We frequently have regrets from the past and worries about the future weighing down our heads amid the hurry of modern life. The only place life really happens is in the present moment, which mindfulness returns us to. This chapter delves deeply into the mindfulness practice and its transforming potential to improve our everyday life.

Essential Mindfulness

The practice of mindfulness involves being totally present in the here and now, conscious of our thoughts and feelings without distraction or judgment. We shall look at:

- **Historically Based:** Origins of mindfulness throughout many spiritual and cultural traditions.
- **Current Adaptations:** How mindfulness has been included into modern health regimens.

Supporting Science of Mindfulness

There is a plethora of evidence that backs up mindfulness. The following sections explore:

- **Neuroscience:** Modifying the structure and operation of the brain via mindfulness meditation.
- **Psychological Benefits:** Its capacity to lower anxiety, despair, and stress.
- **Physical Health:** How mindfulness helps to increase immunity, sleep better, and lower blood pressure.

Intentional Practice

Practices of mindfulness are numerous. Covered will be:

- **Formal Meditation:** Methods for guided, seated, and walking meditations.
- Informal practices are bringing mindfulness into regular tasks like eating, walking, and even working.

- Developing presence in contacts with others to improve relationships is known as mindful communication.

The Mindfulness and Emotional Intelligence

Understanding and controlling our emotions is emotional intelligence. Subjects covered are:

- **Self-Awareness:** Increasing awareness of your emotional states by mindfulness practice.
- Techniques for effective emotion management are known as self-regulation.
- Empathy is the ability to listen attentively to others and so have a deeper comprehension of their feelings.

Rising Above Mindfulness Obstacles

Typical challenges to mindfulness practice are covered, including:

- **Distractions:** Methods of managing both internal and external distractions.

- Tips for keeping up a regular mindfulness practice are included under Consistency.
- **Expectations:** Taking a long view and controlling the want for quick fixes.

Everyday Mindfulness

We'll offer doable tips for incorporating mindfulness into your daily routine:

- **First Things First:** Easy mindfulness exercises to get you started.
- **Building a Routine:** Establishing a time-efficient, durable practice.
- **Mindful Spaces:** Planning spaces that promote awareness.

Special Populations Mindfulness

Adapting mindfulness techniques for other groups, such as:

- **Kids & Teens:** Mindfulness activities appropriate for developing brains.

- **Workplace:** Putting mindfulness programs into place to lower stress and increase output.
- **Elderly:** Modifying mindfulness for ageing and cognitive health.

Techniques for Advanced Mindfulness

For those prepared to take their practice further, we will look at:

- **Retreats:** The advantages of fully immersed mindfulness-based activities.
- Including tai chi and yoga as part of mindful movement.
- Compassion practices are ways of using mindfulness to develop compassion for oneself and other people.

Connection: The Power of Relationships

Our civilization is woven together by human relationships. As necessary for our health as the air we breathe are they. This chapter explores the enormous effects relationships have on our longevity, happiness, and health.

Relationship Biology

We have connection wired in. The interactions that our brains are made to make with other people have profound biological consequences. Subjects covered include:

- **Neurotransmitters:** The impact of relationships on the 'feel-good' chemicals oxytocin and serotonin release.
- **Stress Response:** The physiological repercussions of stress that can be lessened by social support.
- **Immune System:** The fascinating relationship between immune system and social relationships.

Relationship Psychology

Relationships mold our identities and worldviews. Within this section,:

- **Attachment theory:** The value of safe attachments during childhood and their impact on adult relationships.
- How our communities and groups shape our sense of self is known as social identity.
- Interpersonal dynamics is the intricate tango of expectations, limits, and communication in partnerships.

Growing Positive Connections

Building blocks of healthy relationships are mutual support, respect, and trust. Covered will be:

- **Communication Skills:** Skillful approaches to self-expression and listening.
- Strategies for amicably settling conflicts.
- The cultivation of compassion and empathy for others.

The Relational Spectrum

Every kind of relationship in our life matters, from close friendships to casual acquaintances. Issues covered include:

- **Families:** The special dynamics of kinship bonds.
- **Friendships:** The importance of and changes in platonic relationships.
- **Romantic Partnerships:** Managing the Pleasures and Difficulties of Love.

Identity and Community

We feel purpose and belonging when we feel a part of a community. This section addresses social networks and the value of having a supportive social circle.

- **Community Involvement:** Approaches to interact and support your neighborhood.
- **Global Connectivity:** The effects of existing in a more linked, global society.

Depression and Seclusion

Loneliness can be more harmful to health than connection. Our topics will be:

- **Risks to Health:** The effects of ongoing loneliness on the body and mind.
- **Overcoming Isolation:** Actions to Do if You're Feeling Cut Off.
- **Developing New Relationships:** Advice for growing your social network.

Links Online

We now connect in a very different way via technology. In this part, we look at social media's ability to sour connections as well as its function in preserving them.

Virtual Communities: The emergence and function of internet groups in our social environment.

- **Organizing Online Interactions:** Juggling virtual and in-person relationships.

Extra Thoughts

Life events and phases can have an impact on our relationships. Examined will be:

- **Transitions:** How significant life events like retirement, job changes, or migration affect our social networks.
- **Grief & Loss:** Managing a relationship breakup and the grieving process.
- Understanding the many ways connections are created and sustained in different cultures.

Environment: Shaping Your Health Space

Our environment is the backdrop against which our lives unfold. It's where we eat, sleep, work, and play. This chapter examines the profound influence our immediate surroundings have on our health and provides guidance on creating spaces that nurture well-being.

The Impact of Physical Space on Health

The spaces we inhabit can either promote health or contribute to stress and illness. We'll explore:

- **Air Quality:** The importance of clean air and how to improve indoor air quality.
- **Lighting:** How natural and artificial light affects our mood, sleep, and energy levels.
- **Ergonomics:** Designing living and workspaces that support physical health and prevent injury.
- **Creating a Healing Environment**

A healing environment is one that calms the mind and soothes the body. Topics include:

- **Color Psychology:** The effect of different colors on emotional and psychological well-being.
- **Nature and Biophilia:** Incorporating elements of nature into your environment to reduce stress and enhance creativity.
- **Personalization:** Making a space your own with personal touches that reflect your identity and values.

The Home as a Sanctuary

Your home should be a refuge from the chaos of the outside world. We'll cover:

- **Decluttering:** The mental health benefits of a tidy space and tips for decluttering.
- **Safe Spaces:** Creating areas in your home where you can retreat and feel secure.
- **Family Dynamics:** Organizing shared spaces to foster harmony and collaboration.

Workplace Wellness

The design of our workplaces can significantly affect our productivity and health. This section delves into:

- **Office Layout:** The pros and cons of open-plan offices versus private spaces.
- **Break Areas:** Importance of having spaces to rest and recharge during the workday.
- **Work-From-Home:** Setting up a home office that encourages focus and minimizes distractions.

The Role of Technology

While technology has many benefits, it can also impact our health. Topics include:

- **Digital Clutter:** Managing the mental load of digital notifications and online presence.
- **Tech-Free Zones:** Establishing areas in your home where electronic devices are not allowed.
- **Mindful Use of Technology:** Strategies for using technology in ways that support rather than hinder well-being.

Community Spaces

The health of individuals is tied to the health of the community. We'll discuss:

- **Public Spaces:** The importance of parks, libraries, and other communal areas for social well-being.
- **Accessibility:** Ensuring that community spaces are inclusive and accessible to all.
- **Civic Engagement:** Encouraging participation in community design and policy-making.

Environmental Sustainability

Our personal health is interconnected with the health of the planet. This part provides insights on:

- **Sustainable Living:** Practices that reduce your environmental footprint and promote ecological health.
- **Green Building:** The principles of sustainable architecture and interior design.
- **Conservation:** Ways to conserve resources like water and energy in your daily life.

Special Considerations

Different stages of life and circumstances require different environmental considerations. We'll explore:

- **Children's Spaces:** Designing environments that are safe and stimulating for children.
- **Aging in Place:** Adapting environments to meet the needs of older adults.
- **Healing Spaces:** Creating spaces that support recovery from illness or trauma.

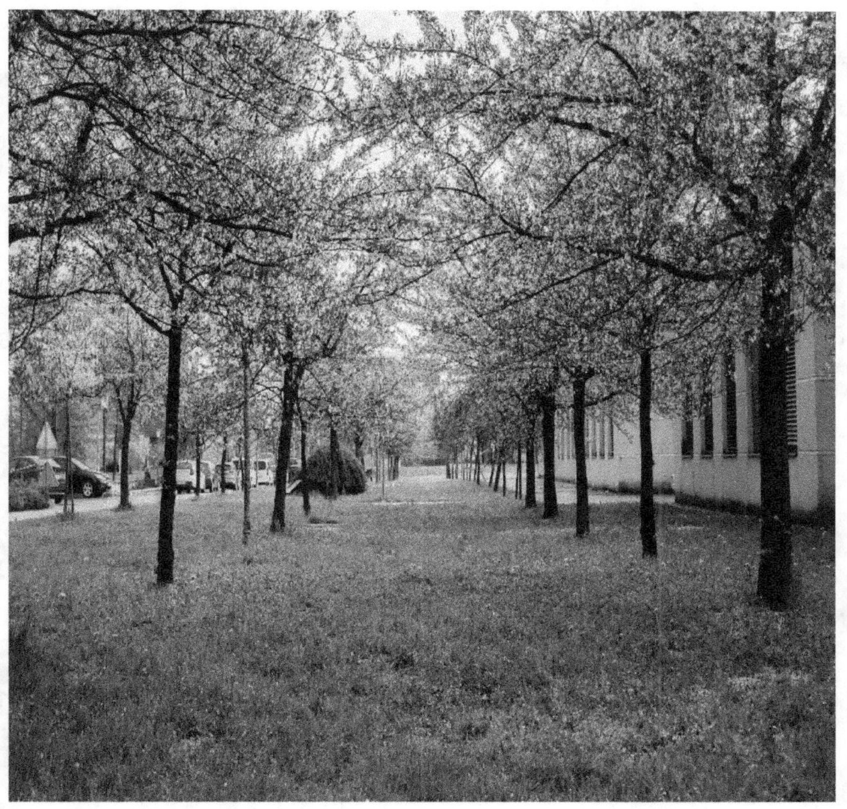

Part III: The 21-Day Livingood Challenge

Preparing for the Challenge

Taking on the Livingood Challenge is an investment in transforming your behaviors and state of health. Success depends on preparation, and this chapter will provide you the information, skills, and attitude you need to maximize this life-altering event.

Making plans

You should know exactly what you want to accomplish before you start. Think back on the reasons you took on this task.

- Want to accomplish what?
- Why will that improve your life?
- Jotting down your goals can help you stay motivated and reminded throughout the challenge.

Knowing the Difficulty

Learn all there is to know about the requirements of the challenge:

- **Daily Commitments:** Actions you must do each day.
- **Anticipated Results:** What you stand to gain from completing the work.
- How to build a network of friends, family, and other challengers for support.

Formulating a Strategy for Achievement

A well-considered plan is your success road map. One aspect of this is defining specific, attainable objectives for the project.

- Making time for difficult activities throughout specific hours of the day.
- Progress tracking is coming up with a plan to keep an eye on your everyday achievements and thinking back on your journey.

Source Collection

Verify that you have all necessary resources:

- Materials comprise any reading, supplies, or instruments required for the task.
- **Information:** Availability of any support groups, applications, or websites.
- **Particular knowledge:** Find experts or mentors who can help when needed.

Nutrition Planning

- To be ready for the task, start by throwing out anything bad from your pantry.
- Shop for nourishing, nutrient-dense foods that meet the requirements of the challenge.
- Preparing Meals Gain fundamental cooking skills to save time and stay on schedule.

Physical Fitness Preparedness

- Do a fitness evaluation to find out where you stand now and to point up any limitations before starting any physical activity.
- Check your equipment to make sure you have the right clothes and gear for your physical activities.
- Workout Routine creating an appropriate exercise regimen that fits your lifestyle.

Psychological Techniques

- To be ready for the task, include deep breathing and meditation into your regular regimen.
- Make a list of positive statements to boost your commitment and self-assurance.
- Identification of stressors and creation of effective stress management techniques.

Practical Points to Remember

- Answer any practical issues that could come up during the assignment.
- Time management is striking a balance among your obligations to your family, job, and social life.

- **Plan Your Travel:** Modify your challenge activities to allow for any travel you may do over the course of the 21 days.
- Backup plans are those in place in case things don't work out as planned.

Allowing flexibility

- Ability to adjust is just as crucial as being ready.
- **Setting and Changing Goals:** Being prepared to adjust your goals when conditions do.
- **Attending to Your Body:** Observing the cues your body gives you and modifying your action as necessary.
- **Maintaining Receptivity:** Be receptive to fresh encounters and educational possibilities all through the challenge.
- Create fresh schedules, try out some healthy behaviors, and start the process of change. Starting down this new route will be both thrilling and difficult this week.

Day 1: Creating the Groundwork

- **Morning Ritual:** To rouse your body and mind, start your day with a glass of water and a few minutes of deep breathing.
- Goal Evaluation Look over your goals again.

Week 1: Kickstarting Your Journey

The first week of the Livingood Challenge is about laying the groundwork for success. It's time to prepare for the challenges and imagine yourself succeeding.

- **Physical Activity:** Go for a vigorous 30-minute stroll to get your circulation flowing.

Day 2: Nutritional Focus.

- **Healthy Breakfast:** Make a nutrient-dense breakfast to fuel your day.
- **Education:** Understand macronutrients and how to balance them in your meals.
- **Mindful Eating:** Practice eating without interruptions, savoring each bite.

Day three: Movement and Mobility

- **Stretching:** Use a 15-minute stretching regimen to increase flexibility.
- **Exercise Exploration:** Try a new type of exercise, such as yoga, swimming, or cycling.
- **Reflection:** Write down how your body feels after moving and stretching.

Day four: Hydration and sleep

Water Intake: Aim to consume at least eight glasses of water every day.

Sleep Hygiene: Create a nightly regimen that encourages peaceful sleep.

Gratitude: Before going to bed, write down three things for which you are grateful.

Day 5: Stress management

- **Breathing Exercises:** Learn and practice a stress-reducing breathing technique.

- **Time Management:** Evaluate your calendar and devise strategies to reduce overwhelm.
- **Relaxation:** Finish the day with a soothing activity, such as reading or taking a bath.

Day 6: Social & Community

- **Connection:** Contact a friend or family member to engage in a meaningful chat.
- **Community:** Take part in a community event or volunteer activity.
- **Support:** Share your challenge experiences with your support group.

Day Seven: Reflection and Planning

- **Review:** Reflect on the week and determine what worked well and what did not.
- Make any necessary changes to your plan for the upcoming week.
- **Preparation:** Plan meals, schedule activities, and establish goals for week two.

Daily Habits

During the week, focus on these everyday habits:

- **Journaling:** Keep a daily record of your food, exercise, and feelings.
- **Affirmations:** Repeating positive affirmations can enhance confidence and motivation.
- **Visualization:** Take a few minutes to visualize your victory in the task.

Week 2: Deepening the Practice

As you approach the second week of the Livingood Challenge, it's important to strengthen the routines you've already begun. This week is about reinforcing the behaviors you've started, investigating them more, and making them a more important part of your life.

Day 8: Intensified Nutrition

- **Whole Foods:** Try to incorporate more whole foods during each meal.
- **Recipe Exploration:** Try making a new healthy recipe with a range of nutrients.

- **Nutrition Journaling:** Keep track of not just what you eat, but also how you feel afterward.

Day 9: Increasing Physical Activity.

- **Activity Variation:** Incorporate a new element into your workout, such as interval training or a different sort of class.
- **Mind-Body Connection:** Try an exercise that combines physical movement and awareness, such as yoga or tai chi.
- **Recovery:** Learn and apply active recovery approaches.

Day 10: Mastering Hydration – Infused Water: Try adding fruits or herbs for diversity

- **Hydration Check-Ins:** Set reminders to monitor your hydration levels throughout the day.
- **Evening Routine:** Avoid drinks that can disrupt sleep, such as caffeine or alcohol, in the evening.

Day 11: Improving Sleep Quality.

- **Sleep Environment:** Make changes to your sleeping environment to increase comfort and relaxation.
- **Relaxation Techniques:** Before going to bed, try a new relaxation method, including progressive muscle relaxation or guided imagery.
- **Sleep Tracking:** If you use a sleep tracker, analyze your data to uncover patterns and areas for improvement.

Day 12: Advanced Stress Management

- **Advanced Breathing:** Use a more advanced breathing technique, such as the 4-7-8 method or alternating nostril breathing.
- **Time Blocking:** Use time-blocking tactics to better manage your day and reduce stress.
- **Leisure Time:** Plan leisure activities that you enjoy and will help you relax.

Day 13: Building Relationships

- **Quality Time:** Spend time with a loved one, focusing on deepening your relationship.
- **Community Service:** Participate in a project that is relevant to you.
- **Expressing Gratitude:** Write a letter of gratitude to someone who has had a good influence on your life.

Day 14: Reflecting and adjusting.

- **Mid-challenge Reflection:** Take some time to reflect on the first part of the challenge. What did you learn? What has been the most challenging?
- **Feedback Loop:** Get feedback from your support network on the changes they've noticed in you.
- **Prepare for Week 3:** Begin planning for the final week, making goals to end strong.

Daily Practices

Continue the daily routines developed in Week 1, focusing on consistency and mindfulness:

- **Journaling:** Continue to journal, concentrating on the depth of your reflections.
- **Affirmations:** Refine your affirmations to reflect your success.

Visualization: Visualize not only the completion of the challenge, but also how you want to sustain these activities after it.

Week 3: Embracing the Transformation

The third week of the Livingood Challenge is a watershed moment in which you begin to accept the transformation that has been occurring. This week is all about consolidating your new habits, reflecting on the changes you've gone through, and getting ready to carry them forward.

Day 15: Celebrating Nutritional Wins

- **Reflection:** Consider how your relationship with food has changed. Celebrate the healthier decisions you have made.
- **Advanced Meal Planning:** Plan your week's meals based on nutrient density and diversity.
- **Sharing:** Share your favorite healthy dish with friends and family.

Day 16: Activity Integration – Introduce new physical challenges, such as a longer trek or advanced fitness class.

- **Consistency:** Consider how your fitness program fits into your daily life.
- **Joyful Movement:** Engage in an enjoyable activity to reinforce the good relationship with fitness.

On Day 17, focus on hydration by drinking water instead of sugary or caffeinated beverages.

- **Hydration Reflection:** Take note of any changes in your energy levels or physical well-being after enhancing your hydration.
- **Water Rituals:** Create 'water rituals' at important intervals throughout your day to keep you hydrated.

Day 18: Sleep Routines.

- **Sleep Quality:** Evaluate the quality of your sleep and make any required changes to your surroundings or habit.
- Consider keeping a dream journal to investigate the relationship between your sleep and subconscious mind.
- **Relaxation Mastery:** Before going to bed, practice a relaxation method that has worked for you before.

Day 19: Stress Resilience.

- **Stress Coping**: Try a new stress-relieving technique, such as writing, art, or music.
- **Support mechanisms:** Assess and strengthen the mechanisms that help you handle stress.
- **Mindfulness Mastery:** Take a longer mindfulness or meditation session to deepen your practice.

Day 20: Deepening Connections

- **Community Engagement:** Take an active role in a community effort or group that shares your ideals.
- **Relationship Building:** Engage in a meaningful conversation with someone new or someone you want to reconnect with.
- Practice gratitude by writing a letter to someone who has helped you through this hardship.

Day 21: Transformation Reflection –

Journey Review: Reflect on the past three weeks and identify the most significant changes in yourself

- **Celebration:** Acknowledge your achievements with a nutritious treat, a self-care activity, or by sharing your success with others.
- **Future Planning:** Set plans for how you will continue to incorporate these habits into your life beyond the challenge.

Daily Practices

In this final week, continue to practice the behaviors you've created, with an emphasis on reflection and integration:

- **Journaling:** Keep a detailed record of your experiences, highlighting your progress and problems.
- **Affirmations:** Use affirmations to reinforce any positive changes you've made.

- **Visualization:** Imagine your future self, fully integrating these new habits into your daily routine.

Part IV: Sustaining Your Habits

Making Health a Lifestyle

Adopting healthy behaviors is only the first step; the real issue is maintaining them over time. This chapter focuses on developing these habits into a lifestyle—a natural and joyful part of your daily life.

Philosophy of a Healthy Lifestyle

A healthy lifestyle is one that prioritizes physical, mental, and emotional well-being. It's about making decisions that prioritize health and pleasure as key values.

Consistency Over Perfection

The key to maintaining a healthy lifestyle is consistency, not perfection. The focus is on creating routines that align with your health goals.

- **Forgiveness:** Being fair to yourself when you make a mistake and getting back on track without judging yourself.
- Flexibility entails adapting your habits to changing circumstances and stages of life.

Integrating Habits into Everyday Life

Make your health routines so ingrained that they are second nature.

- **Consistent Routines:** Incorporate healthy habits into your everyday routines, such as a morning stroll or meditation before bedtime.
- **Environment Design:** Arrange your living and working spaces to promote healthy habits, such as placing a fruit bowl on the counter or a standing workstation.
- **Social Integration:** Include friends and family in your activities to make health a communal experience.

Mindset Shift

A healthy lifestyle begins with an attitude adjustment.

- **Health Identity:** Think of yourself as someone who values and prioritizes health.
- **Positive Reinforcement:** Celebrate your accomplishments and the good sensations that come with healthy living.
- **Continuous Learning:** Maintain your curiosity and openness to new facts about health and wellbeing.

Nutrition: A Way of Life

To maintain a healthy diet, it's important to enjoy preparing and consuming nutritious foods, not merely rely on willpower.

- **Education:** Constantly studying about diet and how it impacts the body.
- **Community:** Share meals and recipes with others to foster a positive food culture.

Active Living

An active lifestyle involves more than just planned exercise. It also includes movement throughout the day, such as climbing the stairs or walking to meetings.

- **Discover Your Passion:** Participate in physical activities you enjoy, making fitness something you look forward to.
- **Rest and Recovery:** Recognize the value of taking rest days and listening to your body's recovery needs.

Emotional Wellbeing

A healthy lifestyle includes maintaining mental health.

- **Stress Management:** Create a toolset of effective stress management practices.
- **Emotional Awareness:** Develop an understanding of your emotions and learn appropriate ways to express them.
- **Support Networks:** Establish solid relationships to provide emotional support.

Lifelong Learning

A healthy lifestyle includes being a lifelong learner.

- **Stay Informed:** Keep up with the most recent health research and recommendations.
- **Experimentation:** Be open to trying new things and changing your habits as you learn.
- **Personalization:** Tailor health information to your own requirements and circumstances.

Overcoming Obstacles and Setbacks

Obstacles and setbacks are unavoidable when attempting to maintain a healthy lifestyle. They are not signals of failure, but rather possibilities for development and learning. This chapter outlines techniques for overcoming these obstacles and maintaining your commitment to health.

Understanding Obstacles

Identifying frequent problems is the first step toward conquering them.

- **Time Constraints:** Challenging schedules might make it difficult to prioritize health.

- **Motivation Fluctuations:** Motivation naturally fluctuates.
- **Environmental Temptations:** Unhealthy choices are frequently more accessible and easy.

Setbacks are stepping stones

Reframe setbacks as stepping stones toward success:

- **Growth Mindset:** Look at obstacles as opportunities to build resilience and flexibility.
- **Lessons Learned:** Analyze what caused the setback and how you might avoid it in the future.
- **Positive Outlook:** Keep a positive attitude and focus on progress rather than perfection.

Strategies for Overcoming Obstacles.

Prepare yourself with practical ways for navigating problems.

- **Planning:** Anticipate potential difficulties and devise strategies to overcome them.
- **Flexibility:** Be open to change your objectives and goals as necessary.
- **Support Systems:** Ask friends, family, or a health coach for help and accountability.

Dealing with Motivational Dips

Motivation dips are typical; here's how to deal with them.

- **Small Goals:** Divide larger goals into smaller, more doable activities.
- **Intrinsic Rewards:** Seek internal delight in healthy behaviors rather than only external outcomes.
- **Variety:** To keep your audience involved, keep your routine fresh and engaging.

Navigating environmental challenges

Your environment can have a significant impact on your habits.

- **Healthy Environment:** Create a setting that promotes your health goals.
- **Mindful decisions:** Be aware of your decisions, especially in challenging situations.
- **Preparation:** Keep healthy options available to avoid temptation.

Emotional Resilience

Building emotional resilience is critical to overcome setbacks.

- **Stress Management:** Learn effective stress-management practices.
- **Emotional Awareness:** Recognize and manage your emotions without engaging in unhealthy behaviors.
- **Coping Skills:** Develop a set of healthy coping strategies for dealing with negative emotions.

Maintaining momentum.

Maintain the momentum, even after a setback:

- **Consistent Routines:** Follow your routines as much as possible.
- **Celebrating Success:** Recognize and appreciate every accomplishment, no matter how minor.
- **Continuous Improvement:** Always seek ways to improve and polish your habits.

Learning From Relapse

If you relapse into previous habits, consider it a learning experience:

- **Self-Compassion:** Show yourself kindness and understanding.
- **Analysis:** Determine what caused the relapse and how to prevent it in the future.
- **Recommitment:** Reaffirm your dedication to your health goals and begin again.

Resources for Continued Growth

Continued growth is vital for maintaining the success you've made on your health journey. It entails a dedication to lifelong learning, adaptability, and the use of numerous resources to further your development. This chapter discusses resources for continued personal and health development.

Lifelong Learning

- Accept the mindset of a perpetual learner.
- **Stay Curious:** Be open to new information and experiences that can broaden your understanding.
- **Educational Opportunities:** Attend health and wellness-related workshops, courses, or seminars.
- **Reading:** On a regular basis, read books, articles, and research papers about health.

Professional Development

Personal health and professional development are inextricably linked.

- **Career Goals:** Establish clear, actionable objectives for your professional progress.[1]. – Continuously study and acquire new abilities to enhance your career and personal life.Build a professional network of persons who share your interest in health and wellbeing.

Online Platforms and Communities

The internet provides a variety of resources.

- **Online Courses:** Platforms such as Coursera provide courses on a variety of topics, including health and wellness.[2].
- **Forums and Groups:** Join online groups to share your experiences, ask questions, and get help.
- **Blogs and Podcasts:** Subscribe to blogs and podcasts that offer great insights and advice for living a healthy lifestyle.

Experienced persons can provide excellent coaching and mentoring

- **Health Coaches:** Consult with a health coach to get tailored guidance and assistance.
- **Mentors:** Find a mentor who exemplifies the healthy lifestyle you want to maintain.

- **Peer Support:** Connect with peers who are also committed to a healthy lifestyle to provide reciprocal encouragement.

Technology and Applications

Use technology to promote your growth:

- **Fitness Trackers:** Use these gadgets to track your physical activity, sleep, and other health data.
- **Mobile Apps:** Get apps for habit tracking, meditation, nutrition, and more.
- **Social Media:** Follow health professionals and influencers for daily inspiration and insight.

Personal Reflection

Self-reflection is an effective technique for improvement.

- **Journaling:** Keep a journal to record your experiences, struggles, and accomplishments.
- **Meditation:** Use meditation to gain clarity and concentration on your growth objectives.

- **Feedback:** Seek feedback from others on a regular basis in order to gain new perspectives on your success.

Community Involvement

Being a member of a community can encourage growth:

- **Volunteering:** Contribute to health-related causes or organizations.
- **Local Events:** Attend local health and wellness events, workshops, and lectures.
- **Advocacy:** Promote health programs that benefit your community.

Work-Life Balance

Maintaining balance is critical for sustainable growth.

- **Time management:** Make time for personal development by prioritizing your tasks.
- **Stress Reduction:** Implement effective stress management practices.

- **Leisure Activities:** Take up hobbies and activities that will revive you and provide a break from your daily routine.

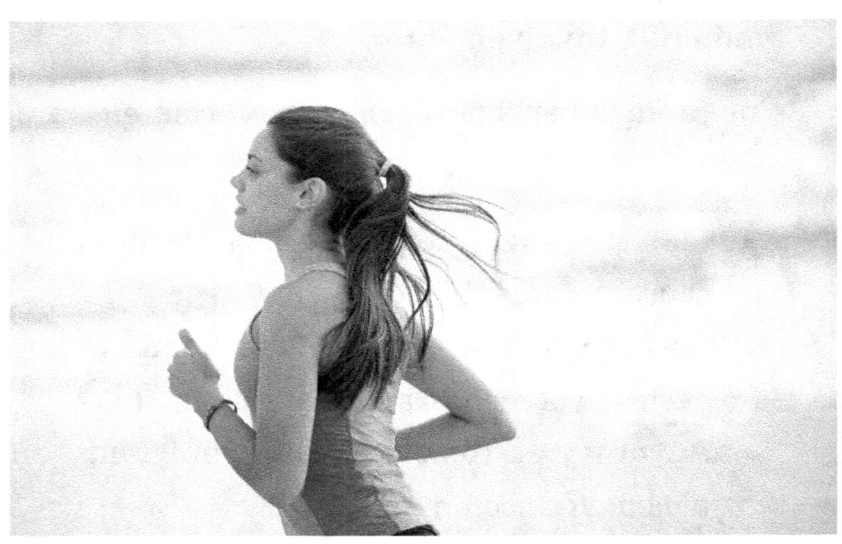

Conclusion

Reflecting on Your Journey

As we near the end of "Livingood Health Habits," it's time to pause and reflect on the journey you've walked. This is more than just the end of a book; it is the start of a new chapter in your life, one centered on your health and well-being.

The path traveled

Consider where you started and the accomplishments you've made:

- **Initial Goals:** Re-evaluate the health goals you established at the start of this trip.
- **Overcome Challenges:** Recognize the challenges you've faced and the perseverance you've demonstrated in overcoming them.
- **Habits Formed:** Recognize the new habits you've developed and the good impact they've had on your life.

Transformational Experiences

Consider the modifications in several areas of your life:

- **Physical Changes:** Keep track of any changes in your physical health, such as improved energy, better sleep, or weight control.
- **Mental and Emotional Growth:** Consider any mental or emotional changes you've gone through, such as decreased stress or increased happiness.
- **Lifestyle modifications:** Consider the modifications you've implemented in your daily routine and how they've led to a healthier lifestyle.

Lessons Learned

Every journey contains essential lessons:

- **About Health:** What have you learned about health and wellness that has surprised or impacted you the most?

- **About You:** How have you evolved personally? What have you learned about your strengths, limitations, and values?
- **For the Future:** What lessons can you apply as you continue to prioritize your health?

Gratitude and acknowledgment

Express thanks for the support and resources that have helped you:

- **Support Networks:** Express gratitude to those who have helped you, such as family, friends, and healthcare providers.
- **Self-Appreciation:** Praise yourself for the time and work you've put into this journey.
- **Resources Used:** Recognize the books, tools, and groups that have provided advice and inspiration.

The Road Ahead

Look ahead to the future with excitement and a plan.

- **Continued Growth:** Explain how you plan to grow and sustain your healthy behaviors.
- **Set New Goals:** Determine new health and fitness objectives to strive for.
- **Lifelong Commitment:** Decide to make health a lifelong quest rather than a fleeting phase.

Final Thoughts

As you conclude this book, realize that the journey to health is never fully complete. It is a continuous process of learning, growing, and adjusting. The habits you've developed and the knowledge you've obtained will serve you well throughout your life. Accept the journey with an open heart and a willing spirit, knowing that each step you take is a step closer to a healthier, happier you.

Next Steps: Living the Livingood Life

As you turn the last page of this guide, you stand on the verge of a new beginning. "Living the Livingood Life" is about maintaining the momentum you've gained and incorporating health and wellness ideas into all aspects of your life.

Revisiting Your Vision

Your desire for a healthier lifestyle was the spark that started this adventure. Revisit and refine that vision.

- **Long-Term Goals:** Establish new long-term goals that are consistent with your vision of health.
- **Life Integration:** Consider how your health goals tie into your overall life goals.
- **Continuous Evolution:** Let your vision change as you develop and learn.

Building on foundations

The foundations you've set are simply the beginning point:

- **Habit Stacking:** Add new, complementing behaviors to those you've already developed.

- **Routine Refinement:** Tweak your routines to improve their efficiency and enjoyment.
- **Lifestyle Assessment:** Evaluate your lifestyle on a regular basis to ensure that it is consistent with your health goals.

Advanced Healthcare Strategies

As you develop, look at more advanced tactics for health optimization:

- **Functional Fitness:** Include exercise that supports your regular tasks and challenges.
- **Nutritional Advances:** Learn more about nutritional research and how to adjust your diet to your specific needs.
- **Mind-Body Techniques:** Learn about advanced mind-body techniques such as Qigong and advanced yoga.

Community and Connection.

A supportive community is crucial for maintaining health.

- **Health Circles:** Form or join groups that focus on health and wellness.
- **Mentorship:** Provide advise to individuals who are beginning their health journey.
- **Social Wellness:** Take part in social activities that promote wellness and happiness.

Lifelong Education

Commit to continuing education in health and wellness.

- **Continued Learning:** Stay up to date on the newest health research and trends.
- **Workshops and Seminars:** Attend activities that provide in-depth insights into health-related issues.
- **Certificates:** Consider getting certificates in nutrition, exercise, or wellness coaching.

Health is a value

Make health a key value.

- **Decision Filter:** Use health as a filter while making life decisions, ranging from work changes to personal relationships.

- **Value Transmission:** Discuss the importance of health with your family and community.
- **Advocacy:** Support health-promoting policies and initiatives.

Adaptability and resilience

Develop the adaptability and resilience required to live a healthy lifestyle.

- **Change Management:** Learn how to negotiate life's transitions while prioritizing your health.
- **Resilience Training:** Develop mental and emotional resilience via techniques such as meditation and journaling.
- **Flexibility:** Be adaptable in your approach to health, changing as needed.

Celebrating Milestones

Celebrate your health milestones:

- **Recognition:** Acknowledge your accomplishments, no matter how minor.

- **Rewards:** Treat yourself to events that reinforce your health values.
- **Sharing Success:** Use your triumphs to encourage and motivate others.

Planning for the future

Look forward and plan for your future health.

- **Preventive Measures:** Prioritize preventive health measures to guarantee long-term well-being.
- **Health Legacy:** Think about the health legacy you wish to leave for your family and community.
- **Sustainable Practices:** Make sustainable health choices that benefit both you and the environment.

Living the Livingood. Life is a commitment to long-term health and enjoyment. It is about making daily choices that improve your well-being. As you continue down this route, keep in mind that each step is part of a greater journey toward a full, fulfilling life.

A Final Note of Encouragement

As you stand on the verge of a new chapter in your life, having read the pages of "Livingood Health Habits," I offer you this final word of encouragement:

Accept the route you've chosen with an open heart and a clear head. The journey to well-being is not straight; it is full of peaks and valleys, each with its own set of lessons and opportunities for progress. Remember that every step forward, no matter how tiny, is a win on its own.

Remember that the habits you've developed are more than just behaviors; they're the seeds from which your future health will grow. Water them consistently, nourish them with encouragement, and allow them to flourish with patience.

Recognize that there will be days when inspiration wanes and the obstacles appear insurmountable. In these moments, think about why you started, how far you've come, and what you still want to accomplish. Allow these to be the beacons that lead you back to your path.

Celebrate your accomplishments, learn from your setbacks, and always strive for balance. Health is more than just the absence of disease; it is the equilibrium of the body, mind, and spirit. Seek this harmony in whatever you do, and let it be the compass that guides your decisions.

Connect with individuals who share your vision for a healthy lifestyle. You may work together to create a supportive community that encourages and inspires. Share your story, listen to others', and find strength in the common goal of well-being.

Remember that you are not alone while living the Livingood Life. There are numerous options available to you, including books, communities, professionals, and more. Use them, learn from them, and let them inspire your journey.

Above all, believe in yourself and your potential to create change. You have the ability to control your health and life. Every day brings new opportunities to live better, love more, and laugh more.

Go out with courage, dear reader. The world is waiting for you to make your mark, live completely, and shine brilliantly. Your road to health is more than a personal success; it is a gift to everyone whose lives you touch.

Live well, live fully, and experience the Livingood Life.

Appendices

Recipes for Health

The path to health is paved not only with good intentions, but also with nutritious meals that nourish the body and satisfy the senses. This appendix has a handpicked collection of recipes that incorporate the health and wellness principles you've learned. Each recipe is intended to be nourishing, delicious, and a tribute to the joys of eating well.

Breakfast Recipes

Begin your day with energy and vitality with these nutritious breakfast options:

1.Superfood Smoothie Bowl

- Blend together the acai berries, banana, and a splash of almond milk.
- Garnish with chia seeds, sliced almonds, and fresh berries.

2. Steel-cut oatmeal with a twist: cook with unsweetened almond milk.

- Add grated apple, cinnamon, and a touch of honey.
- Finish with walnuts and a sprinkling of flaxseed.

Lunch Recipes:

Nourish your midday with meals that are both satisfying and nutritious:

1. Quinoa Salad with Lemon Tahini Dressing

- Combine cooked quinoa, diced cucumber, cherry tomatoes, and parsley.
- Drizzle with a dressing consisting of tahini, lemon juice, garlic, and water.

2. Hearty Vegetable Soup

- Simmer a variety of veggies, including carrots, zucchini, and kale, in a rich tomato broth.
- Season with herbs such as thyme and basil to enhance the flavor.

Dinner Recipes

End your day on a high note with nutritious and delectable dinners:

1. Grilled Salmon with Avocado Salsa Top salmon fillets with a salsa of avocado, red onion, cilantro, and lime juice

- Serve alongside roasted sweet potatoes.

2. Stir-fried Tofu with Vegetables

- Sauté tofu cubes till golden, then set aside.
- Stir fry a variety of veggies, including bell peppers, broccoli, and snap peas.
- Combine the tofu and vegetables in a sauce made with soy sauce, ginger, and garlic.

Snacks and sides

Keep hunger at bay with snacks and sides that are simple but filling:

1. Hummus with Veggie Sticks

- Blend chickpeas, tahini, lemon juice, and garlic to make a smooth hummus.
- Serve with carrots, celery, and bell peppers.

2. Baked kale chips

- Combine kale leaves, olive oil, and a pinch of salt.
- Bake till crispy, then enjoy as a crunchy, nutritious snack.

Desserts

Indulge in sweets while maintaining your health goals:

1. Fruit and Nut Dark Chocolate Bark

- Melt the dark chocolate and spread it thinly onto a parchment-lined tray.
- Before the mixture settles, sprinkle with chopped nuts and dried fruits.
- After it has cooled and set, break it into pieces.

2. Baked Apples with Cinnamon: Core apples and fill with oats, cinnamon, and coconut oil.

- Bake until apples are tender and filling is golden.

Beverages

Stay hydrated and rejuvenated with these healthy beverages:

1. Green Detox Juice

- Juice the kale, spinach, cucumber, green apple, and lemon.
- Consume immediately for a refreshing nutrient boost.

2. Herbal Tea Infusions

- Steep your preferred herbal tea, such as chamomile or peppermint, in boiling water.
- For added flavor, garnish with a lemon slice or a mint leaf.

These recipes are more than just directions for cooking; they are invitations to discover the world of healthy eating. They urge you to explore with different flavors, textures, and ingredients, all while feeding your body and pleasing your palate. As you continue to live the Livingood Life, let these recipes to inspire you to prepare meals that are both healthy and enjoyable to eat.

Daily Habit Tracker

Daily routines are the foundation of long-term health. Consistency is essential, and a daily habit tracker is a helpful tool for preserving it. This appendix includes a complete habit tracker to help you monitor and maintain the good habits you've formed.

Designing Your Habit Tracker

A habit tracker should be adjusted to suit your specific goals and lifestyle. Here's how to design one.

1. Identify Habits: Create a list of the habits you want to track. These could include consuming eight glasses of water per day or meditating for ten minutes every morning.

2. Set Parameters: Determine the frequency of each habit (daily, weekly, etc.) and the optimal time of day to practice it.

3. Create a Template: Create a template that will allow you to simply track when you complete each habit. This could be a real journal, a digital spreadsheet, or a smartphone app.

Use Your Habit Tracker

To get the most out of your habit tracker, consider the following suggestions:

1. Consistent Use: Keep your tracker updated on a regular basis. Some people find it beneficial to do this at the same time every day, such as just before bed.

2. Evaluate & Reflection: At the conclusion of each week, evaluate your tracker. Consider what worked well, what didn't, and why.

3. Adjust as Needed: Use your reflections to make changes to your behaviors or the way you monitor them.

Sample Habit Tracker

Here's a simple weekly habit tracker template that you may use or modify.

Habit	Monday	Tuesday	Wednesdays	Thursday	Friday	Saturday	Sunday
Drink water							
Morning exercise		✓		✓	✓		
Read		✓	✓	✓	✓		
Meditate	✓	✓	✓	✓	✓	✓	✓
Healthy Eating	✓	✓	✓		✓		

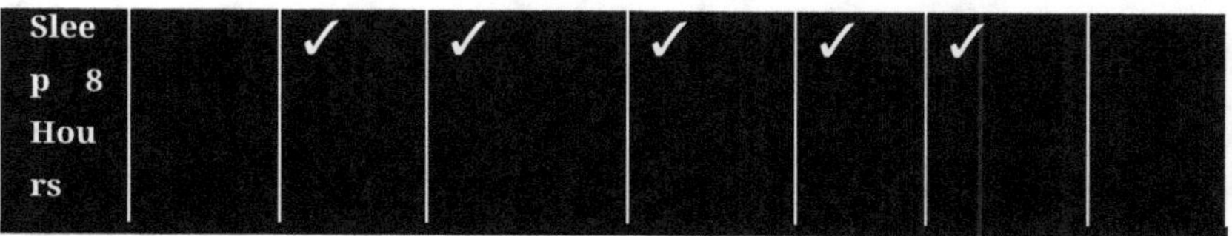

| Slee p 8 Hou rs | | ✓ | ✓ | ✓ | ✓ | ✓ | |

I've left the 'Drink Water' row empty for you to fill in as per your routine. This table provides a clear visual representation of your weekly habits, making it easier to track your progress.

Habit-Tracking Apps

For those who prefer digital options, there are numerous habit tracking apps that include reminders, motivating messages, and progress charts. Some prominent alternatives are:

- **Habitica:** This app turns habit tracking into a game.
- **Loop Habit Tracker:** Provides a simple interface and detailed graphs.
- **Streaks:** Assists you in maintaining long periods of regular habit performance.

A daily habit tracker is more than a tool; it is a mirror that reflects your dedication to your health. It clarifies where you're thriving and where you need to put more effort. Use it as a guide, motivator, and record of your progress in living the Livingood Life.

Frequently Asked Questions

As you follow the ideas outlined in "Livingood Health Habits: The Essential Guide to Everyday Well-Being," questions may emerge. This section is dedicated to answering such questions, offering clarification, and expanding your understanding of a health-conscious lifestyle.

Q: What influenced the title and subtitle of the book?

A: "Livingood Health Habits" was inspired by a desire to live well and feel good every day. The book's holistic approach to health is reflected in its subtitle, "The Essential Guide to Everyday Well-being," which emphasizes that well-being is a daily practice rather than an occasional goal.

Q: How can I establish and maintain long-term healthy habits?

A: Maintaining good health habits over time necessitates a combination of constant practice, personalization, and a supportive environment. It's also vital to recognize tiny triumphs and be patient with yourself because habits take time to develop.

Q: Can I still eat my favorite foods while following the book's recommendations?

A: Absolutely. A balanced approach to nutrition is essential. It is about moderation, not deprivation. Enjoy your favorite meals in moderation, and aim to include a range of nutrient-dense foods in your diet.

Q: What if I miss a day or fall behind on my habits?

A: Missing a day or falling up is a normal part of the process. What really matters is how you respond. Instead of feeling guilty, use it as a learning experience and return to your normal routine as soon as feasible.

Q: How do I deal with social settings that threaten my health habits?

A: Plan ahead of time in social situations, and don't be afraid to bring your own healthy selections or suggest activities that are consistent with your routines. Communicate your health objectives to your friends and family so they can support you.

Is it required to use a habit tracker?

A habit tracker, while not required, is a very useful tool for many people. It gives you a visual depiction of your progress and can serve as a motivator to stay consistent.

Q: How can I keep motivated when I'm not seeing immediate results?

A: Concentrate on the inherent benefits of your health behaviors, such as feeling more energized or sleeping better, rather than the exterior outcomes. Trust the process, and keep in mind that substantial changes take time.

Q: What are some strategies for fitting extra physical activity into a busy schedule?

A: Look for ways to stay active throughout the day, such as climbing the stairs, walking during breaks, or performing brief, high-intensity workouts. Remember that even tiny quantities of activity can accumulate.

Q: How can I keep my healthy habits while traveling?

A: Prioritize hydration while traveling, choose healthy food alternatives when available, and stay active by walking around new sites or visiting hotel gyms. Consider carrying snacks and workout gear.

Q: Can this book help with certain medical conditions?

A: "Livingood Health Habits" is a basic guide to healthy living, but it is not a substitute for professional medical advice. If you have a specific health concern, speak with a doctor for tailored advice.

Q: How will I continue to learn and improve in my health journey after I finish the book?

A: Continue your education by reading additional health-related literature, attending workshops, and keeping up with the most recent research. Engage in health networks, both online and offline, to share your experiences and learn from others.

Your health journey is unique to you, and inquiries are a natural part of the learning process. Use these

FAQs as a starting point, and don't be afraid to seek out additional information as you continue to live the Livingood Lifestyle. Remember that each inquiry you ask is a step toward greater understanding and better health.